CHANGE YOUR BRAIN, CHANGE YOUR AGE
Master Questionnaire

Plus

PREVENTING ALZHEIMER'S RISK ASSESSMENT
Questionnaire

And

AMEN CLINIC MSQ
Memory Screening Questionnaire

Copyright 2012 Daniel Amen, M.D.

Table of Contents

Introduction

Welcome to the Amen Clinics suite of assessment tools to help you change your brain and your age. This set of assessments includes both paper and pencil tests that you will find in this booklet and assessment tools on the web.

Here you will find the Change Your Brain, Change Your Age Master Questionnaire and Answer Key. Dr. Amen's work is based on tens of thousands of brain SPECT scans performed at his clinic. But a long time ago he realized that not everyone is able to get a scan. His books are translated into 30 different languages and if someone reads it in China or Brazil odds are they are not going to get a scan. So, based on thousands of scans, Dr. Amen developed a series of checklists to help predict what a scan would look like, based on the symptoms endorsed. It is not as good or as accurate as a scan, but, in Dr. Amen's opinion, it is next best. Based on how you score the answer key and Brain System Summaries will give you ideas on how to personalize this program for your needs. Of course, you should always talk to your own health care professional.

The Amen Clinic Brain System Summaries give you a quick reference guide to the different ways to optimize the "prefrontal cortex", "anterior cingulate gyrus", "basal ganglia", deep limbic system", temporal lobes", and "cerebellum".

In this program Dr. Amen argues that the best way to decrease your risk of getting Alzheimer's disease is to decrease or prevent all of the risk factors that are associated with it. In the "Preventing Alzheimer's Risk Assessment Questionnaire and Scoring Interpretation" you will learn about your own risk for Alzheimer's disease and other forms of dementia. This will help to lead you to a personalized plan of how to decrease each risk factor you may have.

The "Amen Clinics MSQ: Memory Screening Questionnaire and Interpretation" is a short questionnaire geared to uncover the most common memory symptoms associated with significant brain problems.

The "Preventing Alzheimer's: A Step-by-Step Plan" is a succinct document to give you a head start in developing your own plan to keep your brain healthy as you age.

You will also find information about the Amen Clinics, www.amenclinics.com and Dr. Amen's new online community "The Amen Solution" www.amensolution.com.

But this is only part of the assessment tools available to you. There is a Brain Health Audit on www.amenclinics.com that you can take and a sophisticated 40 minute brain health assessment on The Amen Solution Community Website under our 24/7 Brain Gym.

Knowing the health of your brain is the first step in learning how to optimize it!

CHANGE YOUR BRAIN, CHANGE YOUR AGE
Master Questionnaire

The Change Your Brain, Change Your Age Master Questionnaire will be a great start to helping you evaluate the health and well being of your brain. Plus, it will lead you to specific parts of the program that may be most helpful for you.

Think of this tool as the beginning of making your good brain great and having the best brain possible. For many years I have realized that not everyone is able to get a brain scan to check on the health of their brain. So, in order to bring the life-changing information that I have learned through our imaging work to the most people I have developed a series of questionnaires to help predict the areas of strengths and vulnerabilities of the brain.

Feel free to give these questionnaires to your friends and family members. Brain healthy friends and families are happier friends and families.

A word of caution is in order. Self-report questionnaires have advantages and limitations. They are quick and easy to score. On the other hand, people filling them out may portray themselves in a way they want to be perceived, resulting in self-report bias. For example, some people exaggerate their experience and mark all of the symptoms as frequent, in essence saying, "I'm glad to have a real problem so that I can get help, be sick or have an excuse for the troubles I have." Others are in total denial. They do not want to see any personal flaws and they do not check any symptoms as significantly problematic, in essence saying, "I'm OK. There's nothing wrong with me. Leave me alone." Not all self-report bias is intentional. People may genuinely have difficulty recognizing problems and expressing how they feel. Sometimes family members or friends are better at evaluating a loved one's level of functioning than a person evaluating himself or herself. They may have noticed things that their loved one hasn't.

Questionnaires of any sort should never be used as the only assessment tool. Use this one as a catalyst to help you think, ask better questions and get more evaluation if needed. Always discuss any recommendations with your personal physician.

CHANGE YOUR BRAIN, CHANGE YOUR AGE
Master Questionnaire

Copyright 2012 Daniel Amen, M.D.

Please rate yourself on each of the symptoms listed below using the following scale. If possible, to give yourself the most complete picture, have another person who knows you well (such as a spouse, lover or parent) rate you as well. List other person_____

0	1	2	3	4	NA
Never	Rarely	Occasionally	Frequently	Very Frequently	Not Applicable/known

Other   Self

_____	_____	1.	Trouble sustaining attention
_____	_____	2.	Lacks attention to detail
_____	_____	3.	Easily distracted
_____	_____	4.	Procrastination
_____	_____	5.	Lacks clear goals
_____	_____	6.	Restless
_____	_____	7.	Difficulty expressing empathy for others
_____	_____	8.	Blurts out answers before questions are completed, interrupts frequently
_____	_____	9.	Impulsive (saying or doing things without thinking first)
_____	_____	10.	Needs caffeine or nicotine in order to focus
_____	_____	11.	Gets stuck on negative thoughts
_____	_____	12.	Worries
_____	_____	13.	Tendency toward compulsive or addictive behaviors
_____	_____	14.	Holds grudges
_____	_____	15.	Upset when things do not go your way
_____	_____	16.	Upset when things are out of place
_____	_____	17.	Tendency to be oppositional or argumentative
_____	_____	18.	Dislikes change
_____	_____	19.	Needing to have things done a certain way or you become very upset
_____	_____	20.	Trouble seeing options in situations
_____	_____	21.	Feeling sad
_____	_____	22.	Being negative
_____	_____	23.	Feeling dissatisfied
_____	_____	24.	Feeling bored
_____	_____	25.	Low energy
_____	_____	26.	Decreased interest in things that are usually fun or pleasurable
_____	_____	27.	Feelings of hopelessness, helplessness, worthlessness, or guilt
_____	_____	28.	Crying spells
_____	_____	29.	Chronic low self-esteem
_____	_____	30.	Social isolation
_____	_____	31.	Feelings of nervousness and anxiety

		32.	Feelings of panic
_____	_____	33.	Symptoms of heightened muscle tension, such as headaches or sore muscles
_____	_____	34.	Tendency to predict the worst
_____	_____	35.	Avoid conflict
_____	_____	36.	Excessive fear of being judged or scrutinized by others
_____	_____	37.	Excessive motivation, trouble stopping working
_____	_____	38.	Lacks confidence in their abilities
_____	_____	39.	Always watching for something bad to happen
_____	_____	40.	Quick startle
_____	_____	41.	Short fuse
_____	_____	42.	Periods of heightened irritability
_____	_____	43.	Misinterprets comments as negative when they are not
_____	_____	44.	Frequent periods of deja vu (the feeling you have been somewhere before even though you haven't)
_____	_____	45.	Sensitivity or mild paranoia
_____	_____	46.	History of a head injury
_____	_____	47.	Dark thoughts, may involve suicidal or homicidal thoughts
_____	_____	48.	Periods of forgetfulness or memory problems
_____	_____	49.	Trouble finding to right word to say
_____	_____	50.	Unstable moods
_____	_____	51.	Poor handwriting
_____	_____	52.	Trouble maintaining an organized work area
_____	_____	53.	Multiple piles around the house
_____	_____	54.	More sensitive to noise than others
_____	_____	55.	Particularly sensitive to touch or tags in clothing
_____	_____	56.	Tend to be clumsy or accident-prone
_____	_____	57.	Trouble learning new information or routines
_____	_____	58.	Trouble keeping up in conversations
_____	_____	59.	Light sensitive and easily bothered by glare, sunlight, headlights or streetlights
_____	_____	60.	More sensitive to the environment than others
_____	_____	61.	Snores loudly or others complain about your snoring
_____	_____	62.	Other say you stop breathing when you sleep
_____	_____	63.	Feel fatigued or tired during the day
_____	_____	64.	Feel cold when others feel fine or they are warm
_____	_____	65.	Problems with brittle, dry hair, or thinning hair
_____	_____	66.	Problems with dry skin
_____	_____	67.	Increase in weight even with low calorie diet
_____	_____	68.	Chronic problems with tiredness
_____	_____	69.	Require excessive amounts of sleep to function properly
_____	_____	70.	Difficult or infrequent bowel movements
_____	_____	71.	Morning headaches that wear off as the day progresses
_____	_____	72.	Lack of motivation or mental sluggishness
_____	_____	73.	Feel warm when others feel fine or they are cold
_____	_____	74.	Night sweats or problems sweating during the day
_____	_____	75.	Heart palpitations
_____	_____	76.	Bulging eyes

_____ _____	77.	Inward trembling
_____ _____	78.	Increased pulse rate even at rest
_____ _____	79.	Insomnia
_____ _____	80.	Difficulty gaining weight
_____ _____	81.	Crave sweets during the day
_____ _____	82.	Irritable if meals are missed
_____ _____	83.	Depend on coffee to keep you going/started
_____ _____	84.	Get lightheaded if meals are missed
_____ _____	85.	Eating relieves fatigue
_____ _____	86.	Feel shaky, jittery, tremors
_____ _____	87.	Agitated, easily upset, nervous
_____ _____	88.	Poor memory, forgetful
_____ _____	89.	Blurred vision
_____ _____	90.	Decreased sex drive
_____ _____	91.	Decreased muscle mass and strength
_____ _____	92.	Loss of body hair
_____ _____	93.	Abdominal fat (pot belly)
_____ _____	94.	Decreased bone mass that may lead to osteoporosis
_____ _____	95.	Light sensitive and bothered by glare, sunlight, headlights or streetlights
_____ _____	96.	Become tired and/or experience headaches, mood changes, feel restless, or have an inability to stay focused with bright or fluorescent lights
_____ _____	97.	Have trouble reading words that are on white, glossy paper
_____ _____	98.	When reading, words or letters shift, shake, blur, move, run together, disappear, or become difficult to perceive
_____ _____	99.	Feel tense, tired, sleepy, or even get headaches with reading
_____ _____	100.	Have problems judging distance and have difficulty with such things as escalators, stairs, ball sports, or driving
_____ _____	101.	Night driving is hard
_____ _____	102.	Increased appetite, binge eating
_____ _____	103.	Winter depressions, mood problems tend to occur in the fall and winter months and recede in the spring and summer
_____ _____	104.	Diet is poor and tends to be haphazard.
_____ _____	105.	Do not exercise.
_____ _____	106.	Put myself at risk for brain injuries, by doing such things as not wearing my seat belt, drinking and driving, engaging in high risk sports, etc.
_____ _____	107.	Live under daily or chronic stress, in my home or work life.
_____ _____	108.	Thoughts tend to be negative, worried or angry.
_____ _____	109.	Problems getting at least 6-7 hours of sleep a night.
_____ _____	110.	Smoke or am exposed to second hand smoke.
_____ _____	111.	Drink or consume more than 2 cups of coffee, tea or dark sodas a day.
_____ _____	112.	Use aspartame and/or MSG.
_____ _____	113.	Around environmental toxins, such as paint fumes, hair or nail salon fumes or pesticides.
_____ _____	114.	Spend more than one hour a day watching TV.
_____ _____	115.	Spend more than one hour a day playing video games.
_____ _____	116.	Outside of work time, spend more than one hour a day on the computer.
_____ _____	117.	Have more than 3 normal size drinks of alcohol a week.

CHANGE YOUR BRAIN,
CHANGE YOUR AGE
Master Questionnaire

Answer Key

Place the number of questions you, or a significant other, answered "3" or "4" in the space provided.

_____ 1-10 Prefrontal cortex (PFC) problems, see PFC sheet.

_____ 11-20 Anterior cingulate gyrus (ACG) problems, see AC sheet.

_____ 21-30 Deep limbic system (DLS) problems, see DLS sheet.

_____ 31-40 Basal ganglia (BG) problems, see BG sheet.

_____ 41-50 Temporal lobe (TL) problems, see TL sheet.

_____ 51-60 Cerebellum (CB) problems, see CB sheet.

For the 6 above brain systems, find below the likelihood that a problem exists. If there is a potential problem see the corresponding section of the book or summary sheets.

Highly probable	5 questions
Probable	3 questions
May be possible	2 questions

_____ 61-63 Sleep apnea -- If you answered one or more of these questions with a score of "3" or "4"you may have sleep apnea. Sleep apnea occurs when people stop breathing multiple times at night. It causes significant oxygen deprivation for the brain and people often feel tired and depressed. This condition is best evaluated by sleep study in a specialized sleep laboratory. Treating sleep apnea often makes a positive difference in mood and energy. If you suspect a problem talk to your physician.

_____ 64-72 Hypothyroid -- If you answered three or more questions with a score of "3" or "4"low thyroid issues should be evaluated by your physician. Low thyroid problems can cause symptoms of anxiety, depression, memory problems and mental fatigue.

_____ 73-80 Hyperthyroid -- If you answered three or more questions with a score of "3" or "4"high thyroid issues should be evaluated by your physician. Excessive thyroid problems can cause symptoms of anxiety, agitation, irritability and depression.

_____ 81-89 Hypoglycemia -- If you answered three or more questions with a score of "3" or "4"low blood sugar states should be evaluated by your physician. Low blood sugar or hypoglycemia can cause symptoms of anxiety and lethargy. Eating four to five small meals a day, as well as eliminating most of the simple sugars in your diet (such as sugar, bread, pasta, potatoes, and rice) can be very helpful to balance your mood and anxiety levels.

_____ 90-94 Low Testosterone Levels -- If you answered two or more questions with a score of "3" or "4"low testosterone issues should be evaluated by your physician. Low testosterone levels can cause symptoms of low energy, depression, moodiness, and low libido, as well as the other symptoms. Getting this condition properly diagnosed and treated can make a significant positive difference in your life for both men and women.

_____ 95-101 Scotopic Sensitivity Syndrome -- If you answered three or more questions with a score of "3" or "4"you may have Scotopic Sensitivity Syndrome (SSS). SSS occurs when the brain is overly sensitive to certain colors of light. This can cause headaches, anxiety, depression, problems reading, and depth perception issues. Getting this condition properly diagnosed and treated can make a significant difference for your mental and physical health. To learn more about the diagnosis and treatment of SSS go to www.irlen.com. Most physicians do not know about this disorder, so please do not rely on them for accurate information.

_____ 102 Carbohydrate Cravings -- If you answered this question with a score of "3" or "4"carbohydrate cravings may be a problem. Research has found that some people respond nicely to taking the supplement chromium picolintae, 400-600micrograms a day.

_____ 103 Seasonal Mood Disorder – If you answered this question with a score of "3" or "4"you may have a seasonal mood disorder. Getting outside during daylight hours can be helpful, along with sitting in front of special "full spectrum light therapy" devices for 30 minutes in the morning. See http://www.mayoclinic.com/health/seasonal-affective-disorder/MH00023 for more information.

_____ 104-117 Bad Brain Habit Questions.
For these questions add up your total score, not just the ones you answered 3 or 4.

If you score between 0-6 then odds are you have very good brain habits. Congratulations!

If you score between 7-12 odds are you are doing good, but you can work to be better.

If you score between 13-20 your brain habits are not good and you are prematurely aging your brain. A better brain awaits you.

If you score more than 20 you have poor brain habits and it is time to be concerned. A brain makeover may just change your life!

Amen Clinics Brain System Summaries

The following summaries are a compilation of the work done at the Amen Clinics. Please use this as a reference to understand the different brain systems as they relate to function, problems and treatments.

Executive Brain -- Prefrontal Cortex

Gear Shifter -- Anterior Cingulate Gyrus

Anxiety and Motivation -- Basal Ganglia

Mood Center -- Deep Limbic System

Memory and Temper Control -- Temporal Lobes

Balance and Organization -- Cerebellum

Executive Brain -- Prefrontal Cortex (PFC)

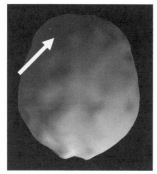
top down surface view

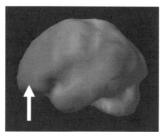
left side surface view

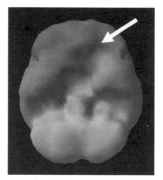
underside surface view

PFC Functions

Attention
Planning
Follow through
Impulse control
Inhibition
Judgment
Empathy
Organization
Morality

PFC Problems

Inattention
Lack of forethought
Procrastination
Impulsive
Disinhibited
Poor judgment
Lack of empathy
Disorganization

Some Conditions Affecting Low PFC Functioning

ADHD   Depression
Brain Trauma   Some dementias
Schizophrenia   Antisocial Personality
Conduct disorders

Low PFC Support

Goal setting   Coaching
Organizational help   Exercise
Relationship counseling Stimulating activities
Higher protein diet   Neurofeedback

Low PFC Medications That May Help

For ADD
    Stimulants such as Adderall, Ritalin/Concerta
    Non-Stimulants: Strattera, Provigil
For Depression
        Wellbutrin
For Psychosis
        Abilify

Low PFC Support Supplements

L-tyrosine, SAMe, green tea, rhodiola, ginseng

Trouble in the PFC is often associated with impulsivity, short attention span, distractibility and difficulties with organization and planning. We have seen a strong correlation between this finding and ADHD and ADD. Low activity in this part of the brain can also be seen with depressive disorders. This pattern has also been seen in response to head injuries affecting this part of the brain, and later in life in some dementia processes.

Gear Shifter -- Anterior Cingulate (AC)

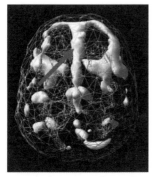
top down active view

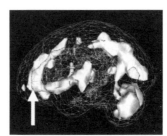
left side active view

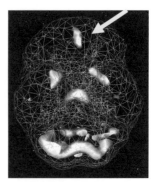
underside active view

ACG   Functions

Brain's gear shifter
Cognitive flexibility
Cooperation
Go from idea to idea
See options
Go with the flow
Error detection

ACG Problems

Gets stuck, Trouble shifting
Inflexible, worries
Holds grudges, oppositional
Obsesses
Compulsions
Argumentative
Excessive error detection
Some forms of addiction

Some Conditions Affecting the ACG

OCD	Anxiety disorders
Addictions	PMS
Eating Disorders	Chronic pain
PTSD	Oppositional Defiant

High ACG Support

Cognitive/behavioral strategies
Intense aerobic exercise
Relationship counseling, anger management
Lower protein/complex carbs diet

High ACG Medications That May Help

SSRIs (Paxil, Zoloft, Celexa, Prozac, Luvox)
Effexor, use XR prep and start slowly
Atypical antipsychotics in refractory cases

High ACG Support Supplements

St. John's Wort, 5HTP, Saffron, Inositol

Increased activity anterior cingulate gyrus activity is often associated with problems shifting attention which may be manifested by cognitive inflexibility, obsessive thoughts, compulsive behaviors, excessive worrying, argumentativeness, oppositional behavior or "getting stuck" on certain thoughts or actions. We have seen a strong association with this finding and obsessive-compulsive disorders, oppositional defiant disorders, eating disorders, addictive disorders, anxiety disorders, Tourette's syndrome and chronic pain. If clinically indicated, hyperactivity in this part of the brain may be helped by anti-obsessive antidepressants or supplements that increase serotonin. Certain forms of behavior modification techniques have also been found to help lessen activity in this part of the brain. When this area is low in activity it is often associated with low motivation and verbal expression.

Anxiety and Motivation - Basal Ganglia (BG)

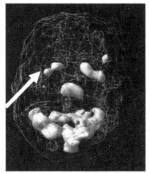 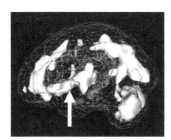 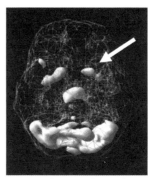

top down active view   left side active view   underside active view

BG Functions

Sense of calm
Sets anxiety level
Motivation
Motor related
Mediates pleasure

BG Problems

Tension, nervousness
Anxiety/panic
Predicting the worst
Tremors/tics
Addictions
Conflict avoidance
No motivation

Some Conditions Affecting the BG

Anxiety Disorders   Tourette's/tics
OCD   PTSD
Movement disorders

High BG Support

Biofeedback   ANT therapy
Hypnosis   Meditation
Relaxing music   Assertiveness training
Limit caffeine/alcohol

High BG Medications That May Help

Antianxiety Meds
    Buspar (buspirone)
Anticonvulsants
Blood pressure meds such as propranolol

High BG Support Supplements

GABA, valerian, magnesium, B6, theanine

Increased basal ganglia activity is often associated with anxiety. We have seen relaxation therapies, such as biofeedback and hypnosis, and cognitive therapies help calm this part of the brain. If clinically indicated, too much activity here may be helped by anti-anxiety medications or supplements may help.

Mood Center -- Deep Limbic System (DLS)

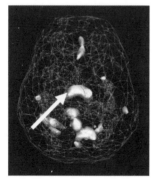

top down active view

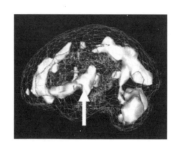

left side active view

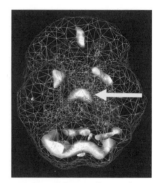

underside active view

DLS Functions

Mood control
Motivation
Attitude
Appetite/sleep
Bonding
Sense of smell
Libido

DLS Problems

Depression
Poor motivation
Poor attitude
Sleep/appetite issues
Tends to isolate
Lack of smell
Negativity, guilt
Hopelessness

High DLS Support

Cognitive-behavioral strategies
Biofeedback, increase left prefrontal activity
Intense aerobic exercise
Relationship counseling
Increased protein diet – The Zone

High DLS Medications That May Help

Antidepressants
   Wellbutrin (buprion)
   Effexor (venlafaxine)
   SSRIs (if ACG present)
Anticonvulsants/Lithium for focal increased activity or cyclic mood changes

High DLS Support Supplements
SAMe, l-tyrosine, DL phenylalanine

Some Conditions Affecting the DLS

Depression   Cyclic mood disorders
Pain syndromes

Increased activity in the DLS is often associated with depression, dysthymia and negativity. It can also be associated with irritability and sadness. In our experience we have seen DLS overactivity can be associated with cyclic mood disorders. If clinically indicated, diffuse increased DLS uptake is often helped by antidepressant medications. If there is also increased anterior cingulate activity consider a serotonergic supplement or antidepressant. If there is not increased anterior cingulate activity consider a supplement, such as SAMe or an antidepressant which increases either dopamine (such as buprion) or norepinephrine (such as imipramine or desipramine). We use anticonvulsants or lithium to help with focal DLS hyperactivity when a cyclic mood clinical pattern is present.

Memory and Temper Control
Temporal Lobes (TLs)

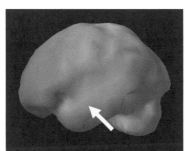

left side surface view

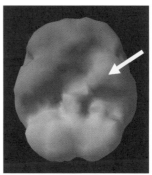

underside surface view

TL Functions	**TL Problems**
Emotional balance	Emotional reactions
Mood stability	Moodiness, irritability
Temper control	Anger, anxiety, fears,
	Phobias, dark thoughts
Memory	Forgetfulness
Language	Trouble finding words
Listening	Processing problems
Reading	Poor reading
Read social cues	Poor social skills
Rhythm, music	Rhythm problems
Spiritual experience	Unusual experiences
Recognize facial	Trouble recognizing
expression	social clues

TL Support
Balanced or high protein diet
Biofeedback to stabilize TL function
Relationship counseling, anger management

TL Medications That May Help
For Mood Stability and Temper Control --
Anticonvulsants, such as Neurontin, Trileptal,
Lamictal, Topamax, or Depakote

For Memory – Aricpet, Exelon, or Namenda

TL Support Supplements
GABA, magnesium, B6

Some Conditions Affecting the TLs
Head injury	Dissociation
Anxiety	Temporal epilepsy
Amnesia	Serious depression
Left side – aggression, dyslexia	
Right side – autistic spectrum disorders	

Abnormal TL (either increased or decreased) activity may be associated with mood instability, irritability, memory struggles, abnormal perceptions (auditory or visual illusions, periods of deja vu), periods of anxiety with little provocation, periods of spaciness or confusion, and unexplained headaches or abdominal pain. Left sided problems are more associated with irritability and dark thoughts, right sided more with anxiety and social struggles.

Coordination and Organization
Cerebellum (CB)

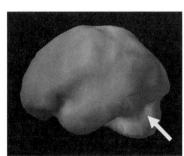

left side surface view

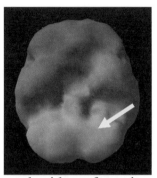

underside surface view

CB Functions

Motor control
Posture, gait
Executive function, connects to PFC
Speed of cognitive integration (like clock
speed of computer)
Organization

CB Problems

Gait/coordination problems
Slowed thinking
Slowed speech
Impulsivity
Poor learning
Disorganization

Some Conditions Affecting CB

Trauma
Alcohol abuse
Autism, Asperger's
ADHD

CB Treatments

Prevention of brain injury
Stop alcohol use or other toxic exposure
Occupational Therapy
Maximize brain nutrition
Coordination exercises, such as dance or table tennis

When the cerebellum is low in activity it has been associated with ADD, autism, brain trauma, toxic exposure, and judgment, disorganization or impulsivity issues.

PREVENTING ALZHEIMER'S
RISK ASSESSMENT Questionnaire

The following questionnaire is based on current scientific research to help you assess your risk for Alzheimer's disease. Once you know your risk you can do things to improve it.

No matter what your age it is important to establish a baseline. It is useful to establish a baseline against which various preventive strategies can be measured, and establishing a baseline allows earlier detection of any disorders that cause memory loss or dementia, which allows them to be treated in their earliest stage to most effectively prevent or delay their progression.

Preventing Alzheimer's Risk Assessment Questionnaire

The following questionnaire is meant as a general screening tool of cognitive function to indicate whether you should consider further testing. Early screening is essential to take full advantage of the preventive and disease therapies that are now available and can mean the difference between living your life without the symptoms of Alzheimer's disease or living out life in a long-term care facility.

The Preventing Alzheimer's Risk Assessment Questionnaire is the first of two self-administered questionnaires that screens for the risk factors associated with Alzheimer's disease. How Is Your Memory screens for its earliest symptoms. As mentioned, questionnaires of any sort should never be used alone as the only assessment tool. Like an isolated laboratory test result, they are not meant to provide a diagnosis. They are simply catalysts to initiate the process of further evaluation when needed. Both of these questionnaires are useful first steps to help determine whether you or a loved one should do further screening. You can find more information and an online Memory Screening Test at www.theamensolution.com.

Please answer the following questions with a yes or no. For every yes answer circle the number provided in parentheses, add your score at the end of the test for interpretation. To give yourself the most complete picture, have another person who knows you well also answer the questions (such as a spouse, partner, child, sibling, parent or close friend or colleague).

Other   Self

_____ _____ 1. (3.5) One family member with Alzheimer's or dementia
_____ _____ 2. (7.5) More than one family member with Alzheimer's or dementia
_____ _____ 3. (2.7) Family history of Down Syndrome
_____ _____ 4. (2.0) A single head injury with loss of consciousness
_____ _____ 5. (2.0) Several head injuries without loss of consciousness
_____ _____ 6. (4.4) Alcohol dependence or drug dependence in past or present
_____ _____ 7. (2.0) Major depression diagnosed by a physician in past or present
_____ _____ 8. (10) Stroke
_____ _____ 9. (2.5) Heart disease or heart attack

_____	_____	10.	(2.1) High cholesterol
_____	_____	11.	(2.3) High blood pressure
_____	_____	12.	(3.4) Diabetes
_____	_____	13.	(3.0) History of cancer or cancer treatment
_____	_____	14.	(1.5) Seizures in past or present
_____	_____	15.	(2.0) Limited exercise, less than twice a week
_____	_____	16.	(2.0) Less than a high school education
_____	_____	17.	(2.0) Jobs that do not require periodically learning new information
_____	_____	18.	(2.0) Within the age range, 65 to 74 years old
_____	_____	19.	(7.0) Within the age range, 75 to 84 years old
_____	_____	20.	(38.0) Over 85 years old
_____	_____	21.	(2.3) Smoking cigarettes for 10 years or longer
_____	_____	22.	(2.5) has one apolipoprotein E4 gene, (if known)
_____	_____	23.	(5.0) has two apolipoprotein E4 genes, (if known)

_____ _____ **Total Score** -- Add up the scores in parentheses for all items checked for self and other.

Interpretation:

If the score is 0 - 3, then you have low risk factors for developing Alzheimer's disease.

If the score is 4-7, then you should do annual screening after age 50 years old.

If the score is greater than 7, then you should annually screen after age 40 years old.

See ways to decrease your Alzheimer's risk and keep the brain healthy with age below.

HOW IS YOUR MEMORY?
Screening Questionnaire

Place a check mark in the columns corresponding to the questions that apply to you or the person you are evaluating. To give yourself the most complete picture, have another person who knows you well also answer the questions (such as a spouse, partner, child, sibling, parent or close friend or colleague).

Severity	Progression	Brain Area Dementia Questions
Yes, Present Now	A Lot Worse Than 10 Years Ago	**TEMPORAL LOBES**
		Is there frequent difficulty remembering appointments?
		Is there frequent difficulty remembering holidays or special occasions such as birthdays or weddings?
		Is there frequent difficulty remembering to take medications or supplements?
		Is there frequent difficulty finding the right words during conversations or retrieving the names of things?
		Are there frequent episodes of irritability, anger, aggression, or a "short fuse" for little-to-no-reason?
		Are there frequent feelings of suspiciousness, paranoia or hypersensitivity without a clear explanation or reason why?
		Is there a frequent tendency to misinterpret what one hears, reads or experiences?
		Temporal Lobe Severity and Progression Totals (add up the total number of checks for this section in each column)
Yes, Present Now	A Lot Worse Than 10 Years Ago	**FRONTAL LOBES**
		Is there frequent difficulty recalling events that occurred a long time ago?
		Is there frequent difficulty with judgments, such as knowing how much food to buy?
		Is there frequent difficulty thinking things through (reasoning)?
		Is there frequent difficulty handling finances or routine affairs that used to be done without difficulty?
		Is there frequent trouble sustaining attention in routine

		situations (i.e., chores, paperwork)?
		Is there frequent difficulty finishing chores, tasks or other activities?
		Is there frequent difficulty with organizing and planning things?
		Are there frequent feelings of boredom, loss of interest, or low motivation to do things that were previously enjoyed.
		Is there a frequent tendency to act impulsively, such as saying or doing things without thinking first?
		Frontal Lobe Progression And Severity Totals (add up the total number of checks for this section in each column)
Yes, Present Now	A Lot Worse Than 10 Years Ago	**PARIETAL LOBES**
		Are there frequent wrong turns or episodes of getting lost traveling to well known places (direction sense)?
		Are there frequent problems judging where you are in relationship to objects around you (for example, bumping into things in a dark, familiar room)?
		Is there frequently a problem recognizing objects just by their feel?
		Are left and right often confused?
		Is there frequent trouble learning a new task or skill?
		Parietal Lobe Progression And Severity Totals (add up the total number of checks for this section in each column)
		Total Progression and Severity Scores

Questionnaire Interpretation

Add your scores in each area and use the key below to determine their meaning.

Severity Score: The number of abilities or behaviors where there is frequent difficulty.
Severity Score = The number of rows where the left column is checked.
Severity Score = _____

Progression Score: The number of abilities or behaviors that are a lot worse than ten years ago.
Progression Score = The number of rows where the right column is checked.

Progression Score = _____

Interpreting The Severity And Progression Scores

A. If both the Severity Score and the Progression Score are 0, then there does not seem to be a problem. Have your partner or significant other verify your answers.

B. If the Severity Score is two or the Progression Score is one and neither of them are three or higher, then there may be an early stage problem or this could be normal aging. If there is any concern about a problem by you or others, then proceed with further testing, such as the memory test found on www.amenclinics.com, the work up described below, or by your physician. An evaluation for depression should also be done if there is any sad mood or loss of motivation. A memory enhancement protocol may be helpful, including: physical and mental exercise to boost nerve growth factors. Avoid any behaviors that increase the risk for a brain injury and take a fish oil to boost the level of omega-3 fatty acids in the brain.

C. If either the Severity Score is three or higher or the Progression Score is two or higher, then the chance of cognitive impairment or dementia is increased. Your memory should be further evaluated by the testing found on www.amenclinics.com, the work up described below, or by your physician. An evaluation for depression should also be done if there is any sad mood or loss of motivation. A memory enhancement protocol may be helpful, including: physical and mental exercise to boost nerve growth factors. Avoid any behaviors that increase the risk for a brain injury and take fish oil to boost the level of omega-3 fatty acids in the brain.

Types of Memory

Memory is a recording of one's experiences stored in the brain – be it an interesting conversation, a piece of information, a "memorable scene," or notable event. There are 3 types of memories differentiated by the time lapse between the experience and the recall of that experience. Each type of memory activates different brain areas when one attempts to recall it.

Working memory resides in the frontal lobe and lasts less than a minute. This form of memory is commonly referred to as one's attention span and lasts up to one minute before being erased. Trying to memorize and dial a telephone number that someone just gave you is an example of working memory.

Short-term memory resides in the medial temporal lobe and lasts a few minutes to a few weeks before being erased. When you try to recall a conversation or a phone number learned a few minutes to a few weeks ago, these brain areas are activated. Not all of one's moment-to-moment experiences activate short-term memory. Only those experiences that are novel, interesting, or those that one intended to remember will sufficiently stimulate nerve cells in the medial temporal lobe to record them.

Long-term memory can last a lifetime. Scientists are not yet certain which brain areas are directly involved in long-term memory. When one tries to recall their first love or the name of a school they went to as a child, they are accessing their long-term memory.

Understanding and Treating Memory Loss

The predominant cause of memory loss is a family of diseases called Alzheimer's Disease and related disorders (ADRD) which includes but is not limited to Alzheimer's Disease, vascular dementia, Parkinson's Disease, and Frontal Lobe dementia. In addition to ADRD, many other conditions cause memory loss. The tables that follow list the major causes of memory loss, the appropriate treatment, and the result of treatment.

Alzheimer's Disease and Related Disorders

Disease	Treatment	Result of Treatment
Alzheimer's Disease	Cholinesterase inhibitor and glutamate modulation	Stabilization and sometimes improvement
Parkinson's Disease	Dopaminergic stimulation	Stabilization and sometimes Improvement
Frontal Lobe Dementia	No established treatment	Not applicable
Vascular Disease	Treat illness and risk factors	Stabilization and sometimes Improvement

Other Causes of Memory Loss and Dementia

Disease	Treatment	Result of Treatment
Anxiety	Anti-anxiety supplements or meds	Improvement
ADHD	Stimulant supplements or meds	Improvement
Depression	Antidepressant supplement or meds	Improvement
Thyroid disease	Thyroid hormone	Improvement
Diabetes	Diet, exercise, meds	Improvement
Metabolic problems	Diagnose etiology and treat	Improvement
Alcohol dependence	Alcohol cessation	Improvement
Drug abuse	Drug cessation	Improvement
Vit. B-12 deficiency	Vit. B-12 replacement	Improvement
Vit. D deficiency	Vit. D replacement	Improvement
Brain infections	IV antibiotics	Improvement

Medications	Adjust medication	Improvement
Fatigue	Diagnose cause and treat	Frequent improvement
Head injury	Cognitive therapy and medication	Frequent improvement
Hydrocephalus	Shunt	Frequent improvement
Cancer	Diagnose and treat	Frequent improvement
Cancer chemotherapy	Brain healthy program	Frequent improvement

Medical Tests to Consider to Evaluate Memory Problems

When a person is suffering from memory problems, the following tests may be useful in evaluating the problem:

Urinalysis
Complete Blood Count
Liver function tests
Folic acid level
Homocysteine level
Vitamin B12 level
25 hydroxy-Vitamin D level
Blood glucose level
Thyroid function tests
Syphilis screening
HIV
Erythrocyte sedimentation
Apolipoprotein E Genotype
Fasting lipid panel
For males, a testosterone level
For females after menopause, an estradiol level
If sleep problems are present, a sleep study to rule out sleep apnea

A brain SPECT study may be helpful if all of the other studies are normal.

KEEP YOUR BRAIN HEALTHY WITH AGE: A STEP BY STEP PLAN

Alzheimer's disease (AD) is no small problem. It currently affects 5 million people in the U.S. and it is estimated to triple by the year 2030. Nearly 50% of people who live to 85 will develop Alzheimer's disease. One of the sad truths is that everyone in the family is affected by AD. The level of emotional, physical and financial stress in these families is constant and enormous. One of the frightening statistics is that an estimated 15% of caregivers of people with AD have it themselves.

Keeping your brain healthy with age requires forethought, a well-researched scientific plan (something that will actually work), and a good prefrontal cortex so that you will follow through on the plan. Here is my five step plan to keep your brain healthy as you age.

Step 1. Know your risk for Alzheimer's disease and related disorders.

See the ALZHEIMER'S RISK ASSESSMENT Questionnaire above.

Step 2. Reduce Your Risk. OK, you have an idea of what risk factors you may have, now, what can you do about it? Here is a list of ways.

Risk: Family member with AD or related disorder or you have the Apo E4 gene.
Reduce: Early screening and take prevention very serious as early as possible.

Risk: Single head injury with loss of consciousness for more than a few minutes.
Reduce: Prevent further head injuries and start the prevention strategies listed below as soon as possible.

Risk: Several head injuries without loss of consciousness.
Reduce: Prevent further head injuries and start prevention strategies early.

Risk: Alcohol dependence, drug dependence or smoking in past or present.
Reduce: Get treatment to stop and look for underlying causes, start prevention strategies early.

Risk: Major depression or ADD diagnosed by a physician in past or present.
Reduce: Get treatment and start prevention strategies early

Risk: Stroke, heart disease, high cholesterol, hypertension, diabetes, history of cancer treatment, seizures in past or present.
Reduce: Get treatment and start prevention strategies early

Risk: Limited exercise (less than twice a week or less than 30 minutes per session).
Reduce: Exercise 3 times a week or more.

Risk: Less than a high school education or job that does not require periodically learning new information.
Reduce: Engage in lifelong learning.

Risk: Sleep apnea.
Reduce: Evaluation and treatment for sleep apnea

Risk: Estrogen or testosterone deficiency
Reduce: Hormone replacement if appropriate

Risk: Work in a hair or nail salon.
Reduce: Make sure there is great ventilation or find a new job. Early prevention strategies are critical to maintaining brain health.

3. Keep your body and brain active

Physical and mental exercise is the best way to keep your brain young. Mental exercise helps the brain maintain and make new connections. Physical exercise boosts blood flow to the brain, improves oxygen supply and helps the brain use glucose more efficiency and helps protect the brain from molecules that hurt it, such as free radicals.

4. Supplements to consider to support healthy brain function

There is a lot of information and misinformation about these substances. Knowing what to do is essential, because some vitamins and supplements work. Dr. Amen takes antioxidants and supplements to keep his brain young and efficient.

High Potency Multiple Vitamin for Brain Health Support

Dr. Amen's Neutraceutical Solutions NeuroVite + – a high potency multiple vitamin and mineral supplement. Very few of us eat the minimum of healthy vegetables and fruits every day - now there's a pharmaceutical-grade supplement that bridges the gap. This formula provides the equivalent of 2-4 servings of healthy fruits and vegetables a day. It is a comprehensive, highly concentrated vitamin and mineral trace element daily supplement containing many nutritional ingredients. It contains a potent antioxidant formula that includes natural beta-carotene, vitamin C, vitamin E, selenium, lutein, lycopene, resveratrol, and the equivalent nutrients of a green apple, tomato, a serving of spinach and broccoli, and 10 grams of dark chocolate.

Fish Oil

Dr. Amen's Neutraceutical Solutions Omega-3 Power is highly concentrated source of health-promoting, omega-3 essential fatty acids from cold water fish to support brain and heart health.

Memory

Dr. Amen's Neutraceutical Solutions Brain and Memory Power was formulated to help support healthy cognitive function by blending ingredients to boost antioxidants, blood flow and acetylcholine in the brain.

Step 5. Eat to Live Long

You are what you eat. Many people are not aware of the fact that all of your cells make themselves new every 5 months. Food is a drug; intuitively we all know this fact. If you have three donuts for breakfast, how do you feel 30 minutes later? Blah! If you have a large plate of pasta for lunch, how do you feel at 2PM? Blah! The right diet helps you feel good. The wrong diet makes you feel bad. Diet is an extremely important strategy to keep your brain healthy with age.

The best diet is one that is low in calories (calorie restriction is associated with longevity), high in omega three fatty acids (fish, fish oil, walnuts and avocados), and antioxidants (vegetables). The best antioxidant fruits and vegetables according to the US Department of Agriculture include: prunes, raisins, blueberries, blackberries, cranberries, strawberries, spinach, raspberries, Brussels sprouts, plums, broccoli, beets, avocados, oranges, red grapes, red bell peppers, cherries, and kiwis. Eat your fruits and vegetables! Your mother was right.

This five step plan is simple and effective. Your brain controls everything you do! Love, honor and respect your brain. Your mental health and longevity depend on it.

Lasting Health Starts with Our Children

Many of the risks for AD occur in childhood. If we are sincere about keeping our brains healthy with age we must start with our children. The ApoE4 gene increases the risk of AD. Having this gene plus a head injury increases the risk further. Many head injuries occur in childhood, especially when playing contact sports or doing other high risk activities. If children are allowed to engage in these activities I think they should first be screened for the ApoE4 gene. If they have it, we should be more cautious with their heads. Children with ADD and learning problems often drop out of school, leaving them at higher risk for dementia. Making sure we properly diagnose and help these children is essential to helping them become lifelong learners. The seeds for depression occur in childhood. Depression often is a result of persistent negative thinking patterns. School programs should be developed to teach children how to correct these patterns, which could help decrease depression. Childhood obesity leads to adult obesity. Educating children on nutrition and exercise can have lifelong benefits. To address these issues, Dr. Amen has developed a high school course, Making A Good Brain Great, to start brain health efforts as early as possible.

ABOUT AMEN CLINICS

Amen Clinics, Inc. (ACI) was established in 1989 by Daniel G. Amen, MD. ACI specializes in brain health plus innovative diagnosis and treatment planning for a wide variety of behavioral, learning, and emotional problems for children, teenagers, and adults. ACI has an international reputation for evaluating brain-behavior problems, such as attention deficit disorder (ADD), depression, anxiety, school failure, brain trauma, obsessive-compulsive disorders, aggressiveness, cognitive decline, and brain toxicity from drugs or alcohol. Brain SPECT imaging is performed at ACI. ACI has the world's largest database of brain scans for behavioral problems.

ACI welcomes referrals from physicians, psychologists, social workers, marriage and family therapists, drug and alcohol counselors, and individual clients.

Amen Clinics, Inc., Southern California
4019 Westerly Place, Suite 100
Newport Beach, CA 92660

Amen Clinics, Inc., San Francisco
1000 Marina, Suite 100
Brisbane, CA 94005

Amen Clinics, Inc., DC
1875 Campus Commons Dr.
Reston, VA 20191

Amen Clinics, Inc., Pacific Northwest
616 120th Ave NE, Suite C 100
Bellevue, WA 98005

www.amenclinics.com
1-888-564-2700

Amenclinics.com is an educational interactive brain website geared toward mental health and medical professionals, educators, students, and the general public. It contains a wealth of information to help you learn about our clinics and the brain. The site contains over three hundred color brain SPECT images, hundreds of scientific abstracts on brain SPECT imaging for psychiatry, a brain puzzle, and much, much more.

View over three hundred astonishing color 3-D brain SPECT images on:
Aggression
Attention Deficit Disorder, including the six subtypes
Dementia and cognitive decline
Drug Abuse
PMS
Anxiety Disorders
Brain Trauma
Depression
Obsessive Compulsive Disorder
Stroke
Seizures

THE AMEN SOLUTION ONLINE PROGRAM

The Amen Solution Online Program will give you all the tools you need to get smarter happier, thinner, and look and feel younger! The Amen Solution is NOT a diet; it is a program to get control of your brain and body for the **REST OF YOUR LIFE.**

The community is dedicated to helping you will **lose weight (if you want to), improve your memory and boost your mood.** You'll also: **elevate your energy, sharpen your focus and calm your anxiety.** And the crazy thing is that all of this will happen when you put into practice the same 10 very simple brain-based solutions.

The program includes:

Detailed questionnaires to know your BRAIN TYPE and personalize this program to your own individual needs. You will also and learn how to decrease your risk of Alzheimer's disease.

Interactive daily online brain and food journals to track your important numbers, calories, and brain healthy habits, like sleep and exercise – THIS IS THE SINGLE MOST IMPORTANT TOOL FOR IMPROVING YOUR HEALTH. If you take 5 minutes a day and keep these journals research suggests it will double your weight loss in just 10 weeks.

Hundreds of brain healthy recipes, tips, shopping lists, and menu plans.

Exclusive, award winning 24/7 BRAIN GYM where you can test, work out and strengthen your brain to reduce stress, improve your memory and attention, and boost your mood. It is like having a personal trainer for YOUR OWN BRAIN. The brain gym has been described as "wildly fun…the positive thinking exercises have carried me through the day…."

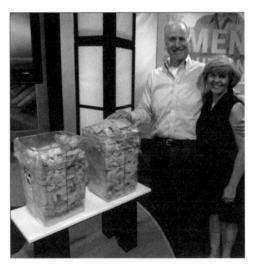

Daily tips and text messages to help you remember your supplements and stay on track to get healthy NOW (if you want).

A relaxation room to decrease anxiety and boost your mood.

Plus much, much more.

One of our patients said after 10 weeks her sister thought she had a mini-face lift.

Another lost 46 pounds with no effort by using the 10 steps.

Sign up at www.theamensolution.com